Contents

Chapter 1

Calisthenics

What comes to your mind when you think of calisthenics?
It can be defined as a form of training involving the use of bodyweight exercises to help build the body muscles. It includes practices such as push-ups, dips, pull-ups, or even pistol squats. It is usually associated with agile and lean athletes and involves mastering your body and developing body balance, control, strength, flexibility, coordination, mobility etc. And it is usually drafted with the athlete's work-out plans.

In simple terms, calisthenics is a form of art which involves using the body weight to use human power as well as athletic ability to its maximum potential. It helps to master control over moving or lifting your body in space. It's a long-practised art and has the name coined from two Greekwords; *kallos*, meaning beauty and *sthenos*, which means strength.

Recently the practice has taken on a new flavour in the form of Competitive Calisthenics; also called street sport or street work-out. This form has seen international light in the form of acrobatics, dance and gymnastics.
The beautiful thing is the fact that it is the most straightforward type of exercise, and does not require fancy instruments.

How calisthenics works

The art of calisthenics involves a gradual transformation of the entire body, physically, emotionally. It is the use of the whole body without emphasizing any muscle over the others. It provides you with a surge of strength from your fingertips down to the bottom of your feet. It is all about the movement of the body in space; hence it is the highest form of "functional movement training". Now functional movement training can be defined as the art of training in such a way that will enhance the method you use for your day to day life tasks directly; it can also be defined as a specific physical requirement needed for your sport or work.

To do this effectively there are some hacks; for instance, it is advisable you make use of elevated surfaces for changing the exercise angles, as well as to increase the percentage of your body weight as you lift it. Also, you can make use of walls and poles (vertical surfaces) to give your body new challenges to overcome and hence build your core.

Chapter 2

What calisthenics can do for you?

These are the things calisthenics can do for you

It increases the strength of the body and provides endurance:

The course of training, the bodyweight is used to exercise specific muscles of the body. In exchange, the tissue becomes more robust and well able to carry your body weight, this is because it is a form of resistance training and as such helps increase the average expenditure of energy. It helps to build body endurance which allows you to hold certain positions for a more extended period and also to perform more reps or sets.

It strengthens mental health:

Another enjoyable truth about calisthenics is the fact that it not only benefits the athlete's body but also benefits the mind; this is because the knowledge of your body's capability leads to proper enlightenment as well as help boost your confidence. It also helps to reduce depression symptoms as it gives the mind something to do hence uplifting one's mood. And then there's also the fact that Calisthenics work-out helps to release endorphins an excitement hormone which relieves stress and tension.

It helps to improve the biomechanics of the body:

Calisthenics helps to improve body balance and coordination. It aids the development of the body all-round, including your body posture. Hence it aids motor coordination and also body balance.

It is easily affordable:

Yes, that's right, calisthenics is a very affordable form of art as it does not require the use of any expensive machinery; it just needs your body and a suitable place to carry out your exercises. You also do not need a gym membership to carry out Calisthenics training; you just need a playground (can also be in the corner of your house), a mat, pull-up bar and gloves (optional).

It is a complete body work-out:

Nearly all Calisthenics training requires a lot of muscles, whether pull-ups which require your arms, core, back, shoulders and chest. This way, you target more muscles (about 2-3 times) than when using machines in the gym.

Can be performed everywhere:

This is another lovely point to note about calisthenics, the world becomes your gym. You can train anywhere as long as you have enough space to carry out the exercises easily. This way, you don't have to worry about getting up early in the morning to go to a gym to carry out your training exercises.

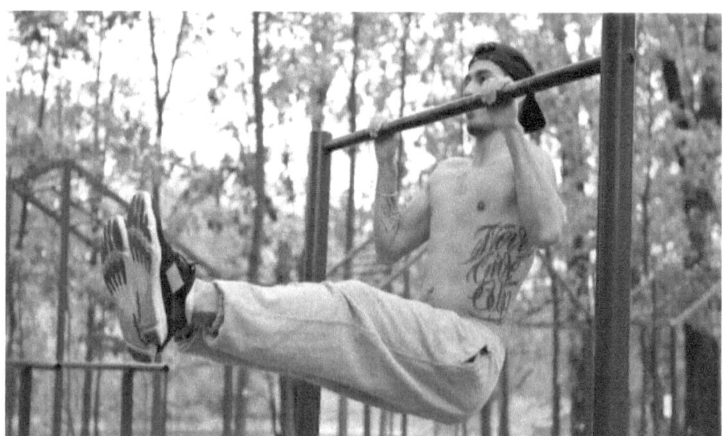

Chapter 3

Before beginning your calisthenics work-out, it is essential to prepare first by warming up. A warm-up helps to prepare the body for the work-out exercises as it loosens the joints of the body; it also helps to increase the flow of blood to your muscles. These actions prepare your muscles and also help to prevent injury during workout.

So in this chapter we will be looking at routines to follow for effective warm-up before your exercise.

1. Rope jumping: you could attempt this by doing your regular rope jump and then alternating between your legs, knees,
2. Running on a spot or around can help too.
3. Swinging your arms round in circles, you can swing both arms at the same time or separately.
4. Scapula Pulses: to do this stand straight with arms stretched out perpendicular to your body, taking a T-form, and then slowly move your arms back and forth.
5. Forward and Backward Scapula Swing: placing your elbows together in front of you, touch your shoulders with your hands and slowly draw circles while retracting your scapula forward and backwards.
6. Scapula Push-up/Pull-up: Either of them is done depending on if you want to do push-ups or pull-ups. Now for this, you should get into a push-up/pull up position, keeping your arms straight and retracting just your scapula.
7. Shoulder Dislocation: for this, you need a resistance band. Stretch the band between your arms while keeping your arms straight. Next, transfer your hands to your back passing over your head all the way down to below your bum.
8. Pulling Band Apart: Still using the resistance band, hold both ends in each hand, push out your chest and retract your scapula. Then place your arms in front of your body and then pull the resistance band apart and towards your chest.
9. Wrist Stretch: put your hands forward with your arms straight

while sitting on your knees, next move your hips in a back and forth sync.

10.   Shoulders Openers: Place your knees on the floor and raise your bum by 90° angle. Next place your arms forward stretching it away from your head and then keep your head as close as possible to the ground.

For your warm-up routine to be effective, ensure you maintain these positions for as long as you can, using a timer to see how your endurance level is.

Chapter 4

Advice on reps, sets and rest on calisthenics

The process of becoming an expert in the world of fitness can be tasking, it is one that demands an enormous amount of time, and it can also drain one. There's need to understand the concepts associated with fitness that is considered to be most valuable. In the field of fitness, the key concepts that you should look out for are,

> a. The Reps,
> b. The sets
> c. Rest
> d. Tempo.

The Reps:

This is used to refer to the number of repetitions. It is used to describe the variable contained in the fitness equation that must be adapted to quickly.

To obtain a maximum result, it is advised that you vary the number of reps and ensure you keep a personal journal to keep records of your progress. Let's look at the following categories:

> a. 1-5 reps: this is commonly used to gain maximum strength. It would help you reach your maximum potential strength-wise. It is usually about 85% of your 1RM (1 rep maximum), in any exercise you do. So, this is not advised for beginners or novice until your form is good enough.
> b. 6-8 reps: this is a standard rep range which is designed to achieve a lovely balance between your strength and also your muscular gains. This category falls around 79-84% of your 1RM. Also requires proper form and perhaps a partner to work with, this can also be an excellent fit for the ladies as it can be mixed with your other set routines to get a perfect body form as ladies.
> c. 9-12 reps: This is the most normal rep range, and is placed around 70-78% of your 1RM. It would allow for optimal

development of your muscles.

d. 13+ reps: Best for novice or beginners as it helps to develop proper form and also to control movements appropriately, and involves anything below 70% of your 1RM.

The Sets:

This refers to the number of times a particular exercise is repeated for the set number of exercises. If for instance, you intend doing 3 sets of 10 reps, it means doing 10 push-ups, or squats then you rest, you do another 10 push-ups and rest again, and finally, you do the third round of 10 push-ups then you rest. That's how it works.

It is important to note that it is equally important to vary your sets, for a beginner between 3-6 sets per exercise is more than enough to achieve a consistent result.

The more reps you do, the fewer the sets you should undertake, hence the categories below can help you in terms of rep: set ratio,

13+ reps: 2-3 sets

9-12 reps: 3-4 sets

6-8 reps: 3-5 sets

1-5 reps: 4-6 sets

It is important to note that the number of reps and sets others can do might not work for you; you have to determine yours. The best way to do this is exercise until you feel your muscles fatigued; this way, you build more strength. So start by working utilizing your base level strength, begin with light exercise for more reps, and do harder exercise for fewer reps. Take a rest, 30 secs or more, after each set to recover and do better in the next sets.

The Rests: this refers to the time interval taken to rest and recover between each set.

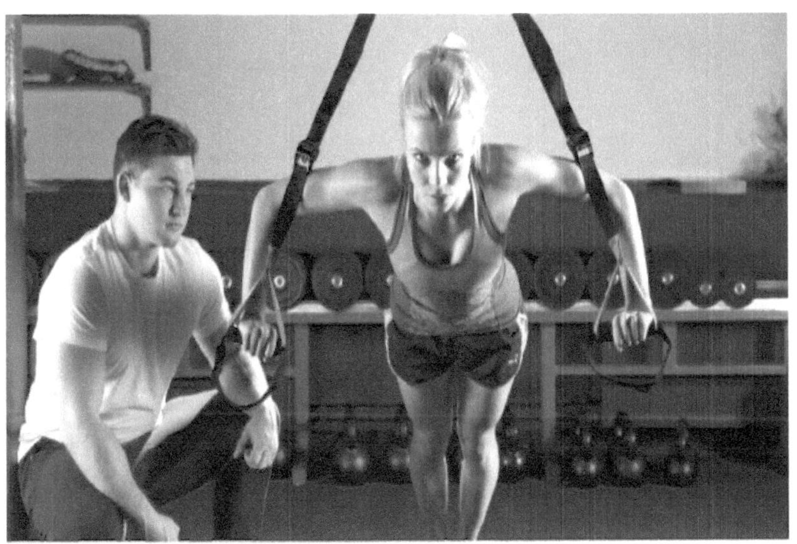

Chapter 5

Nutritional advice that will assist you on your calisthenics workout

Starting a calisthenics fitness program is best done when it is combined effectively with the right nutrition. This way, you are sure of seeing the expected results gradually, and this can motivate you to practice more.

Calisthenics work with diet and its diet program is much less complicated as against the usual norm when it comes to dieting. So it is easy to carry out.

Calisthenics diet plan.

The same way calisthenics exercise is uncomplicated and straightforward, that's how straightforward calisthenics diet is. You can quickly tell if what you're eating is right for your body, or if the food weight is correct. The diet plan is flexible and easily adjusted to suit your fitness goals.

So here are some things you can keep in mind as regards dieting:

a. Firstly, ensure you get rid of all junk food, empty carbs or even processed food within your reach. This includes cereals, soft drinks, sweets, cakes, processed foodstuff, cookies, and pasta, drinks high in sugar, etc. doing this would help regulate your appetite and keep the level of glucose low.
b. Limit eating window. Intermittent Fasting (IF) is a phenomenon common amongst calisthenics athletes. It involves putting a limit on food consumption time to 8 hours only in a day (with exception to water, tea or coffee). This way, your focus is more on nutrient-rich food than junks, which automatically implies that you would consume fewer calories which can result in negative energy balance and so leads to loss of weight.
c. Another secret involves eating lots of food containing fewer calories and also high in fiber, such as veggies and fruits, to give your body the required number of vitamins and minerals.

   d. Food such as lean protein, dairy and grains would be attractive options too.

Calisthenics Supplements

So it is possible you feel you're not getting enough nutrients from what you're eating and you want additional supplements to incorporate in your diet, then you should add

   a. BSCAA this support the muscle mass you've gained, also it helps in building more muscle

   b. Creatine this helps in building as well as recovering muscle mass.

   c. Multivitamins- As always, they are highly important in building your general health as well as your immune system. It includes Vitamin C, D, B complex, etc.

So, in summary, a perfect calisthenics diet would do the following for you:

   a. Control your appetite: it would help provide you with enough discipline when it comes to food; this is because it would keep your blood sugar low and equally constant.

   b. Help gain muscle: eating the right food at the right time does a lot in helping to build muscle faster as well as reduces recovery time, thus giving you a well-defined body.

   c. Keeps you lean: is another beautiful advantage, reducing/limiting the kind of carbs you take in goes a long way.

Importance of diet in calisthenics

   a. First, it helps to provide energy to those who need it.

   b. It can help in reducing weight (weight loss), or body fat, this can be done quickly by cutting down on carbohydrates and fats.

   c. Cutting down on carbs alongside an increase in protein would go a long way to heal the muscles so they can form again.

Chapter 6

Achieving Flexibility

As an athlete, flexibility is highly important as it determines your body's capability to carry out your bodyweight exercises effectively. In this chapter, we'll look at what flexibility is and a list of things to do to ensure your body is flexible.

So what is flexibility?

Flexibility refers to your body's joint and muscles ability to adjust to any position you try to take, and it is an essential element when you consider your physical health. However, while kids are naturally flexible, flexibility reduces as a person grows old, and then you often feel stiff.

Importance of flexibility

1. Stretching your muscles will help release the tension on the muscles and thus make it much easier to move about from place to place.
2. It can also help to improve your body posture.
3. A stretched and flexible body experiences less pain on the back, neck or the shoulders.
4. Reduces risk of injury as you carry out your work-out activities.
5. Another importance is that flexibility makes it possible to move your joints to any average direction.

How to increase flexibility

a. Use of stretching:

Stretching is one of the ways you can improve your body's flexibility. It is often called a warm-up or cool-down activity and very important for your daily routine. It's equally important because it helps to increase blood flow around the body, and ensures your joints are better equipped to carry out the tasks for the day.

How to stretch effectively

Stretching can be done in a variety of ways, but it is highly necessary to keep the following points in mind when stretching.

- Ensure you evenly stretch out both sides,
- You should stretch in such a way that you feel it, but it doesn't hurt you, and you should hold for about 30 secs or more.
- You can tailor your stretch also to the specific activity you're carrying out.

b. Exercises: Some exercises have been designed to aid and improve the body's flexibility, exercises such as tai chi, pilates, yoga, resistance training (e.g. weight lifting). These exercises would help increase your flexibility and also strengthen your body muscles and joints.

Chapter 7

In this chapter, we'll be looking at different exercises that we can do without the need for equipment, as our definition of calisthenics described. And to do this, we'll be looking at the part of the body it is aimed at strengthening.

BACKS

1. **Pull Up**:

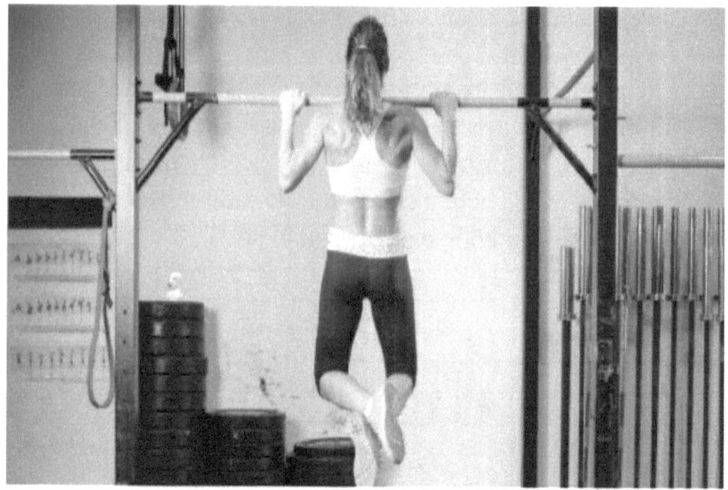

- For this, you would need a bar attached probably to your door frame or position somewhere in your garden.
- Grip the bar using both hands and facing the hands away from you, place your shoulder hip-width apart.
- Pull yourself up and down slowly.

2. **Chin Up:**

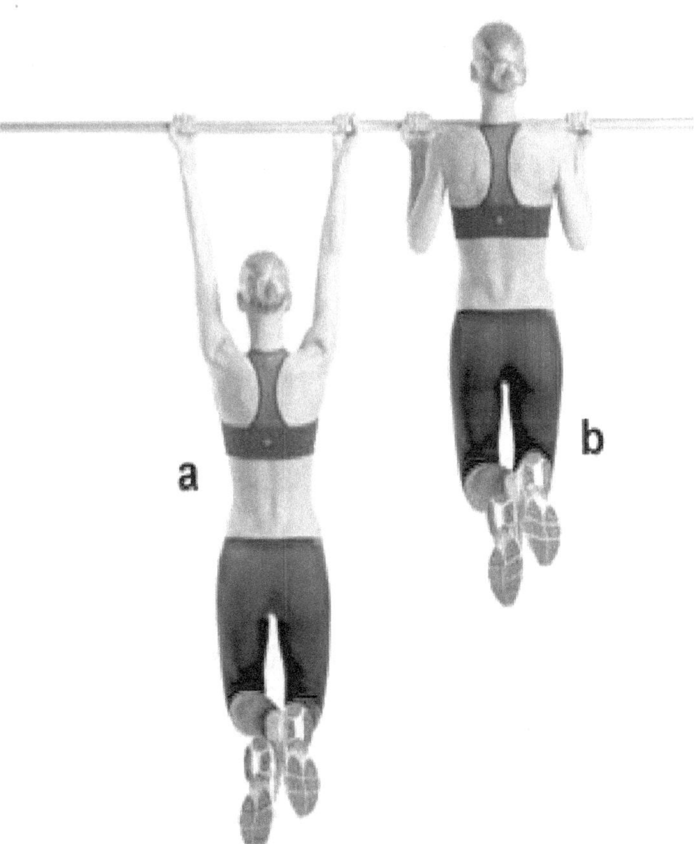

- Maintain the initial stance of the push-up, but the difference is that your hands should be facing you not away from you.
- Also, place the hands closer than in pull up.
- Now slowing pull yourself up.

3. Dynamic:

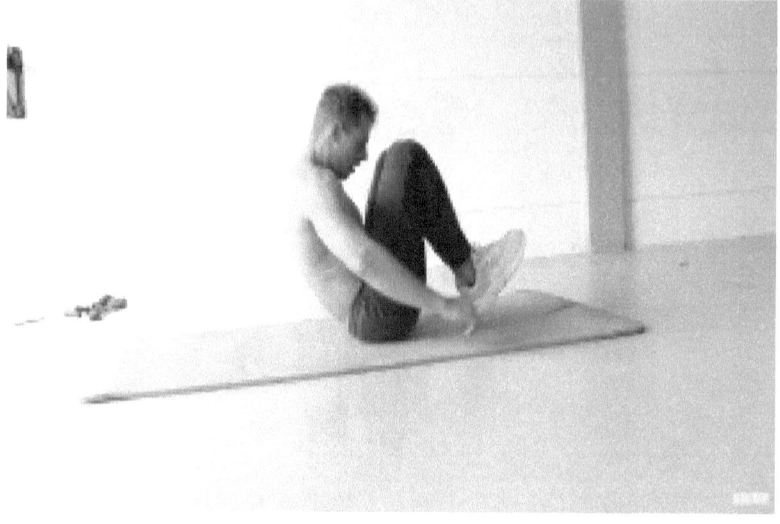

- Lie face up on the mat.
- Bend your knee while raising it up and then lift your back, so your head touches your knee, and you're sitting on your bum,
- Hold that position for a while.

4. Back Extension:

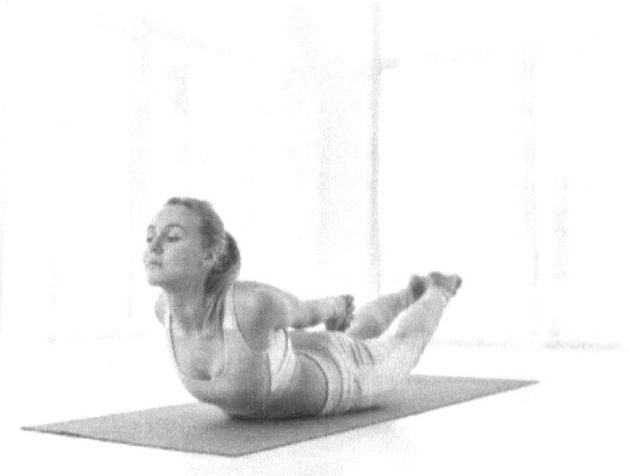

- First lie flat on the ground, ensuring your feet is flat, and your knee is bent slightly.
- Now slowly lift your bum off the floor and placing your back

on the same line with your thighs.
- Try to maintain the position for some time.

5. **Lower Back (Cobra) Stretch**:

- Lie face down on your mat,
- Now push your body up using your arms, while leaving your hips and legs flat on the floor.
- Maintain this position for a while.

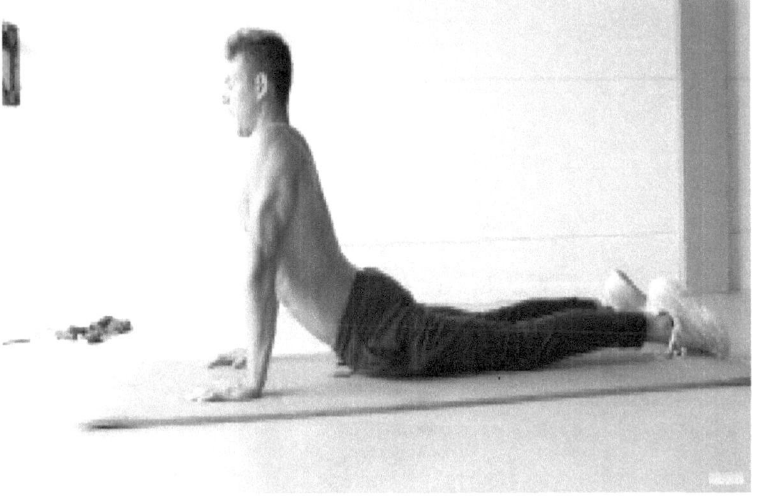

Chapter 8

LEGS

6. Single-leg deadlift

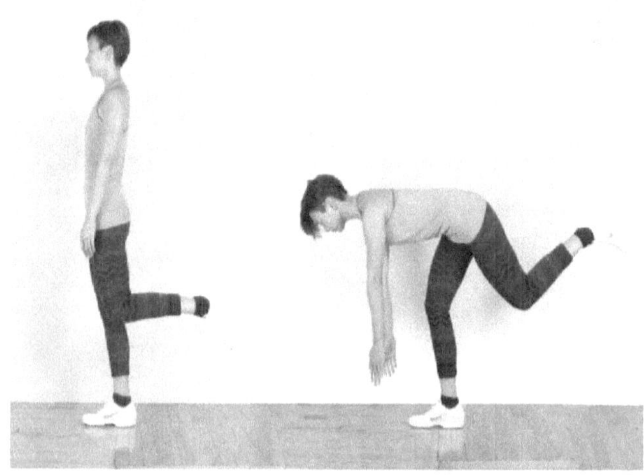

- To do this, start with a standing position with your feet placed together.

- Slightly lift your right leg, after that lower your arms and torso and raise your right leg behind you also.

- Ensure your left knee is bent slightly while reaching your arms as close as possible to the floor.

- Lastly, raise your torso while lowering your right leg.

- Now switch your legs.

7. Squat:

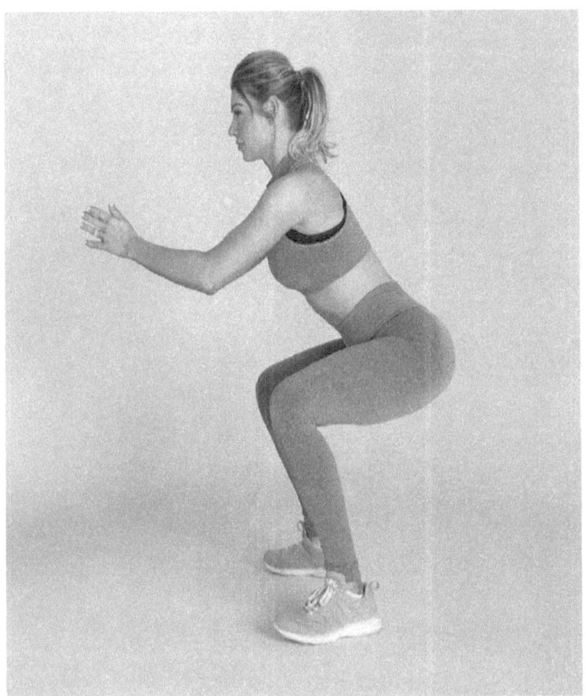

- Begin by standing with your feet turned out by 15° or parallel, whichever position is comfortable for you.
- Slowly start to squat, bending your hips and knees. Do this until your thighs are in a parallel position to the ground.
- While doing the above tasks, your heels must not rise off the floor, when you're done, press your heels to return to a standing position.

8. Pistol squat:

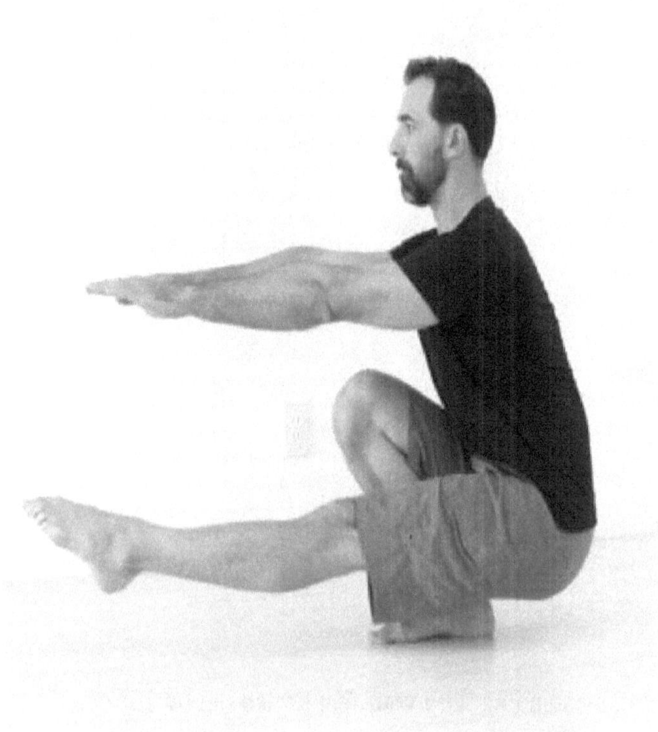

- Hold your arms stretched out straight in front of you.
- Your right leg while flexing your right ankle and also pushing your hips backwards.
- Next, lower your body and keep your right leg also raised, hold still for a while and then return to a standing position.

9. Squat reach and jump

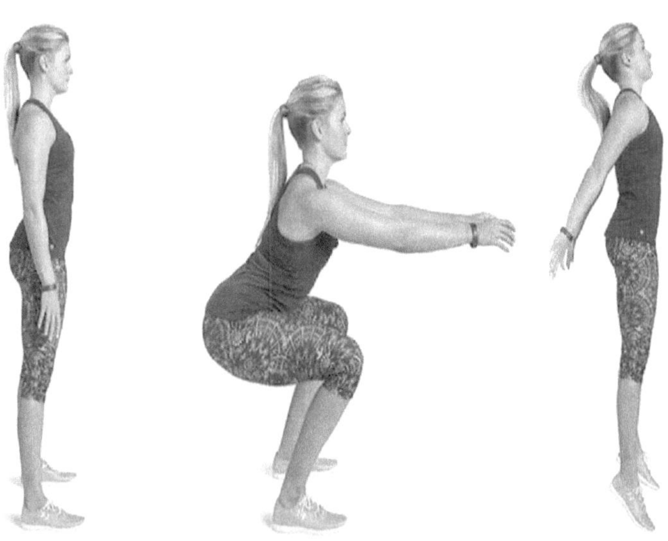

- Start with a normal squat,

- Jump up immediately and reach your arms straight over your
  head.

- Do a couple of reps, take a break and then begin the next set.

10. Chair Pose squat

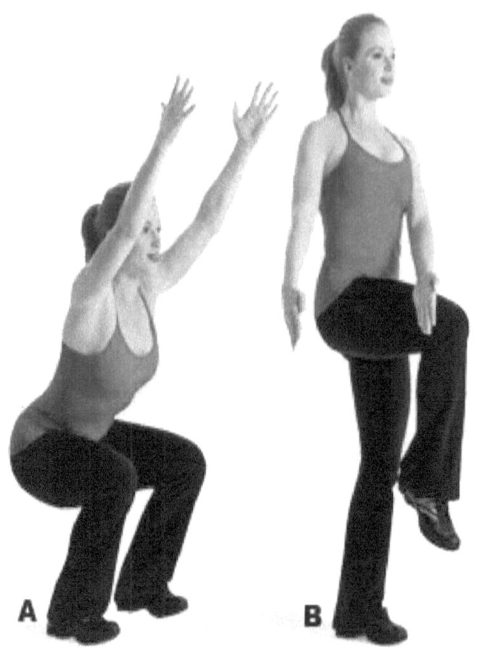

- Start by standing, placing your feet hip width apart and swing your arms up.

- Begin squatting until your thighs are parallel to the ground

- Hold your legs straight and then lift the right knee, ensure you swing your left arm outside your right knee.

- Go back to standing position and then repeat, using the left leg.

11. Wall sit:

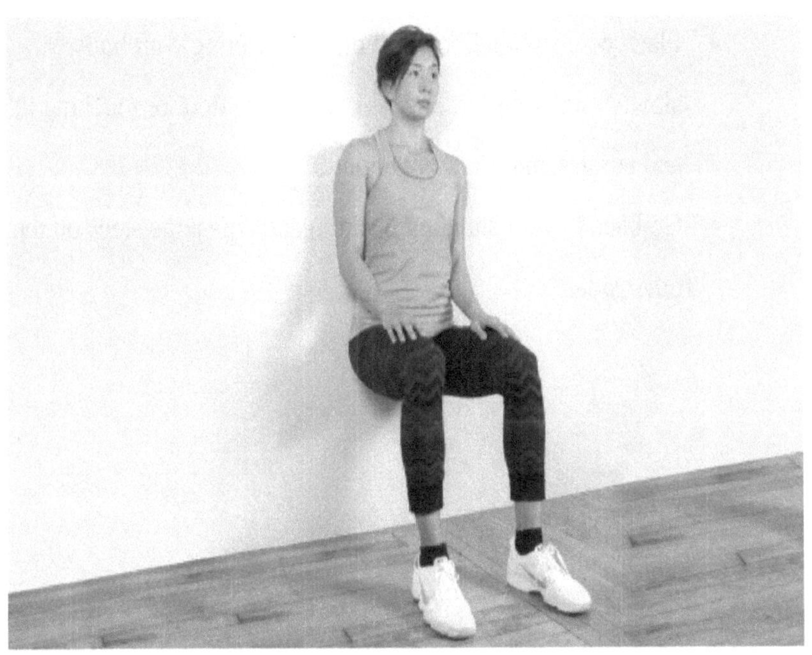

- Stand against the wall and slowly slide your back along the wall. Do this until your thighs are positioned parallel to the floor.

- Ensure your knees are above your ankles directly and also keep your back straight against the wall.

- You can apply 60 secs per sets, or however long you think it would take.

12. Lunge

- Stand placing your hands on your hips and place your feet hip-width apart.

- Place your right leg forward before lowering your body slowly until your left knee is close to the floor or touching it, and at the same time bent about 90°.
- Go back to your standing position and repeat the steps on the other side.

13. Lunge to row:

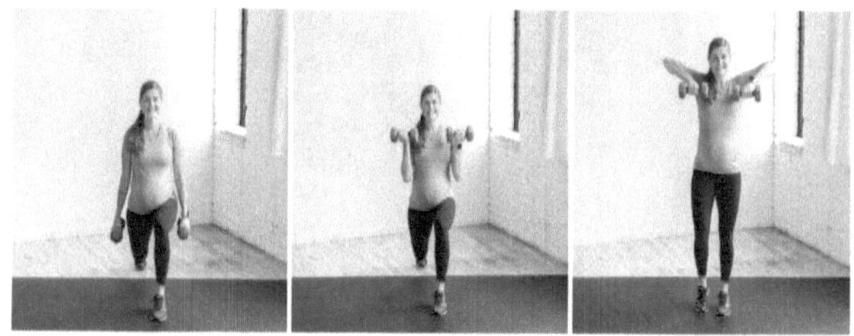

- Begin by making the regular lunge.
- But instead of putting leg back to its starting position at the end of a lunge, lift it from the floor and raise your arms over your head.
- Leave the leg bent at about 90°. You can add weight to bring the heat.

14. Calf raise

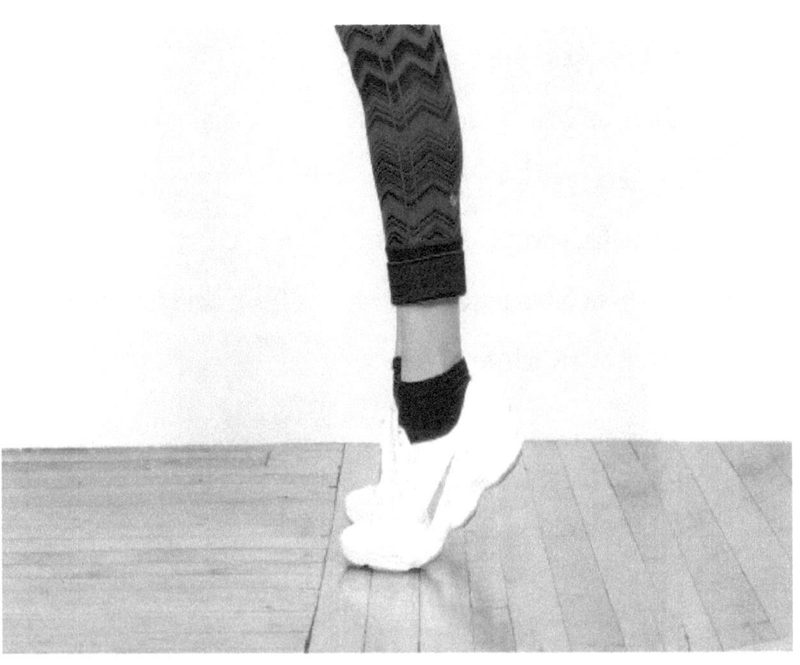

- Take up a standing position and then slowly raise your toes, while keeping your knees straight and your heels away from the floor.
- Hold that position briefly and then come back down. Repeat the process.
- You can also try standing in an elevated position to achieve a wide range of movement.

15. Quadruped leg lift

- Begin on your hands and your knees, flatten your back and

tighten your core.

- Raise up your left leg towards the back until it gets to your hip level and keep it straight,

- Hold that position for as long as you can

- Lift your bottom right toe from the floor, hold for a while and then switch your legs.

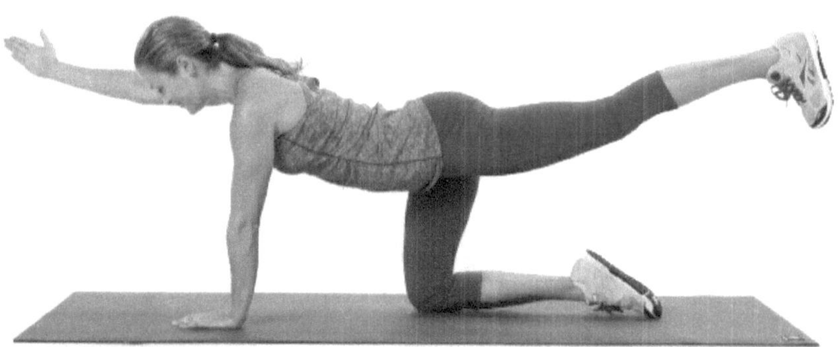

Chapter 9

FULL BODY

16. **Tuck jump**:

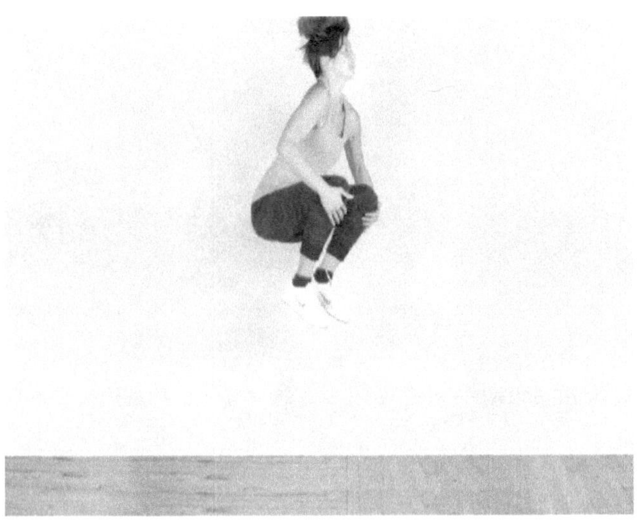

a. Take a standing position while bending your knees slightly.

b. Take a high jump; go as high as possible for you.

c. Bring your knees closer to your chest and extend your arms forward.

d. Land with your knees still bent a little and jump again, repeat the motion again.

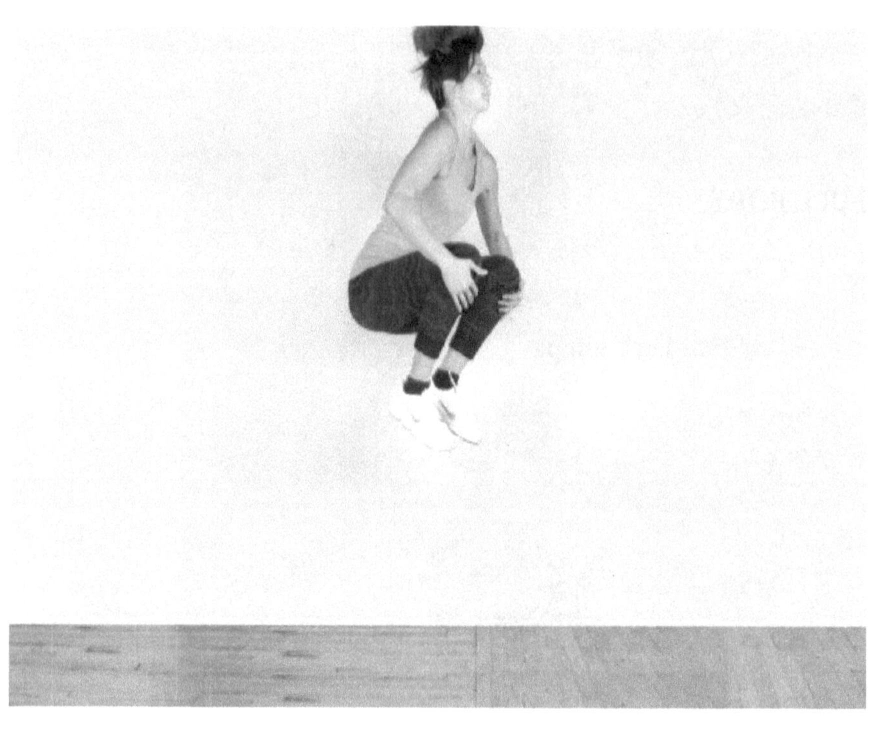

17. Bear crawl

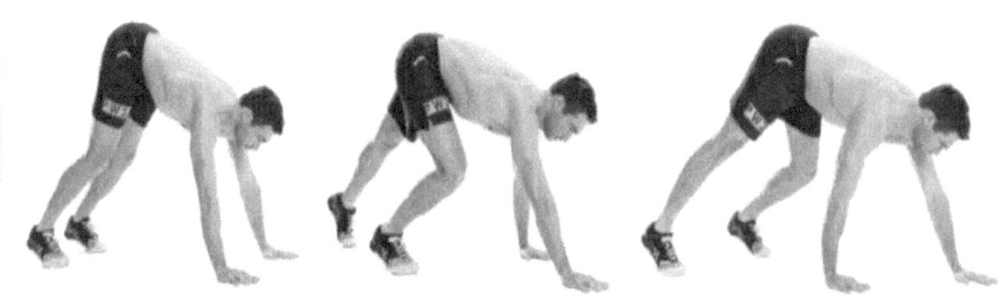

a. Begin on your hands and knees and raise your body onto your toes while increasing the pressure on your core.

b. Now reach forward slowly using your right arm and your right knee, and then move your left hand and left knee.

c. Continue crawling doing 8-10 reps and then rest.

18. Mountain climber

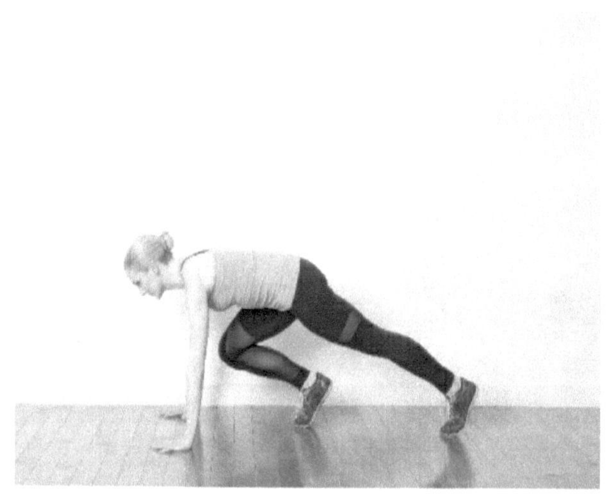

a. Place your weight on your hands and knees, just like the bear crawl

b. Move your left foot forward until it is under your chest directly, at the same time, strengthen your right leg.

c. Next jump and switch legs, this should be done while still keeping your hands on the floor with core tightened.

19. Inchworm

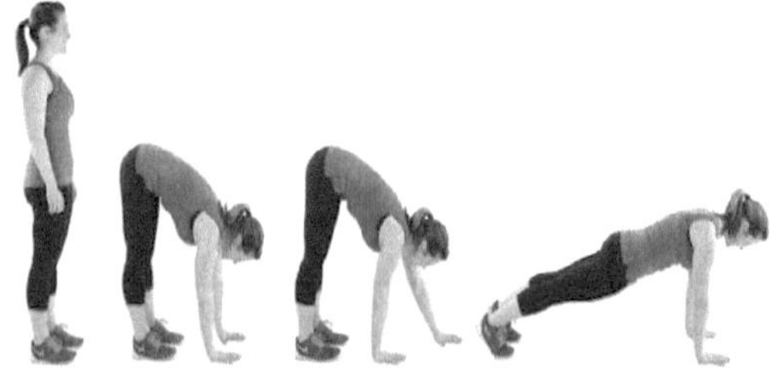

a. Take a standing position and ensure your legs are straight, and knees unlocked.

b. Lower your upper bodies slowly towards the floor then walk your hands forward.

c. After getting to a push-up position, move your legs forward slowly until your feet meet your hands.

d. Walk your hands forward again and move your feet towards your hands as before. Continue this for 5-6 reps before taking a break.

20. Prone walkout

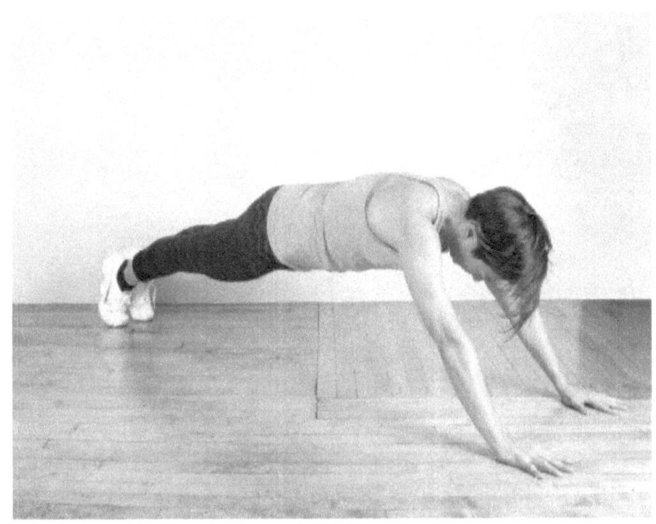

a.   Start by supporting your body weight on all four limbs.

b.   Walk with your hands forward, without moving your toes.

c.   Walk with your hands back to the original position; ensure
     you maintain your balance and stability.

21. Stair climb with biceps curl

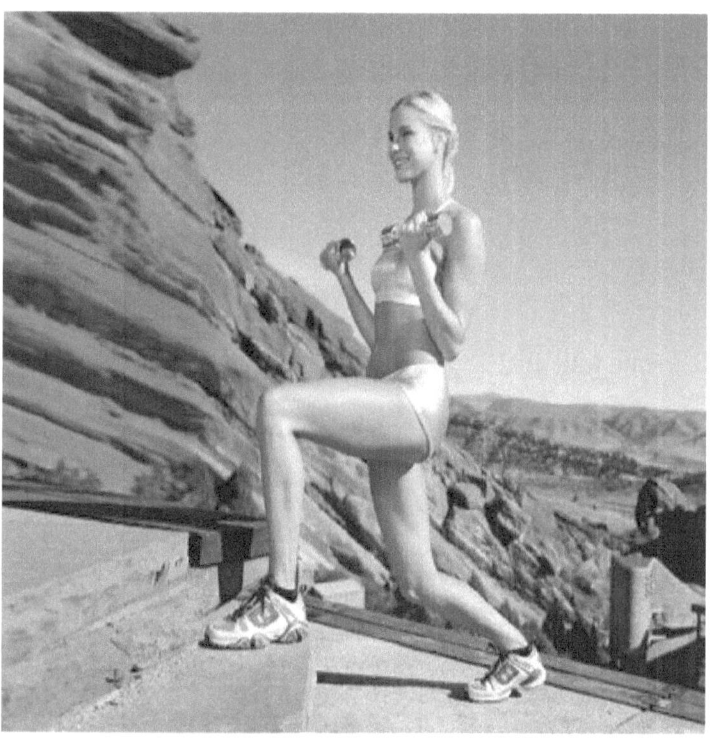

a.   For this, you would need your stairs.

b.   Using dumbbells or any household object with weight, walk
     briskly up and down the stairs.

c.   Also, while doing that, simultaneously do biceps curls to work the whole body.

22. Burpee:

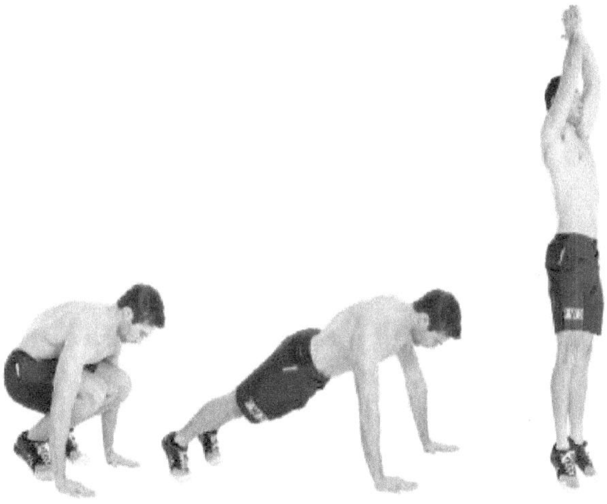

a. Take a low squat position with your hands on the ground.

b. Move your feet back into a push-up pose.

c. Do a complete push-up and return feet to a squat position.

d. Take a high leap up and squat back down while returning to the push-up stance.

23. Plank

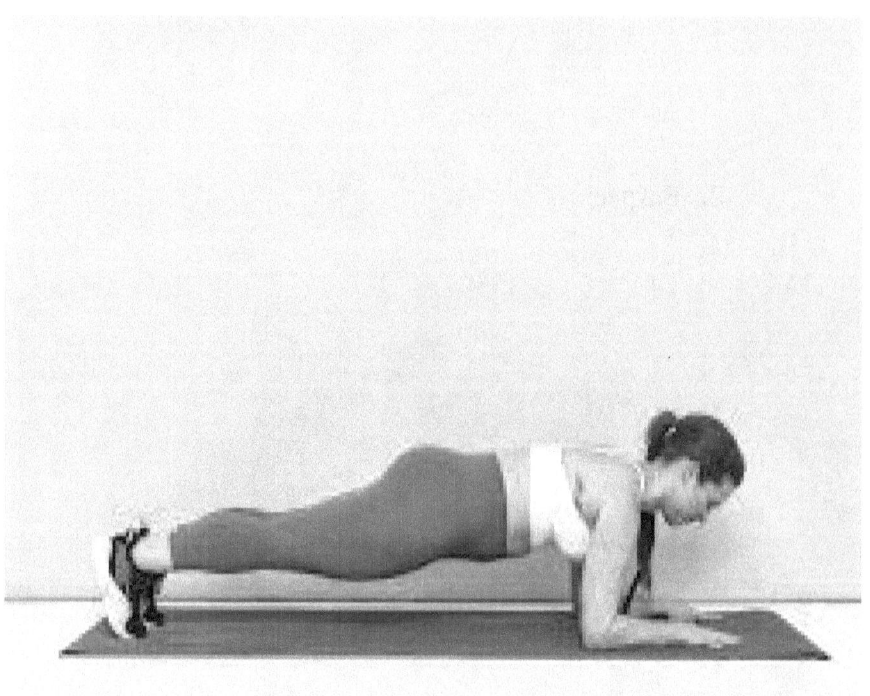

a. Lie facedown placing your forearms on the floor and clasp

your hands together.

b. Now move your legs behind you and raise your body on

your toes.

c. Straighten your back, while tightening your core.

d. You can hold this position for about 30-60 secs, depending

on your endurance level.

24. Plank to push-up

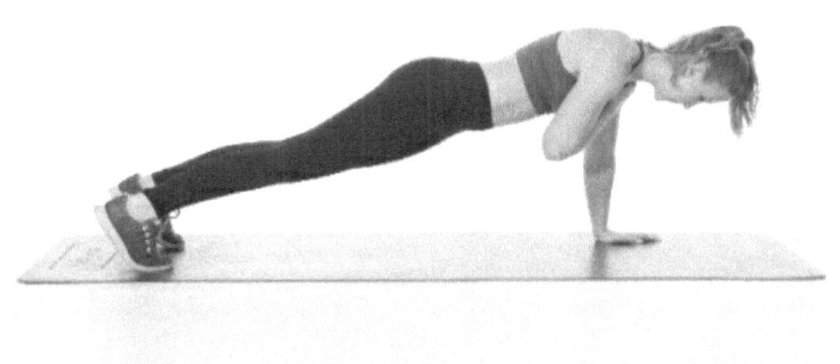

a. Begin with a plank position.

b. Keep one hand on the floor at a time and use it to lift the

body into a push-up position, holding your back straight and engaging your core.

c. Use the one arm to move back into the plank position.

d. Continue the motions alternating the arm from time to time.

Chapter 10

25. Contralateral limb raises.

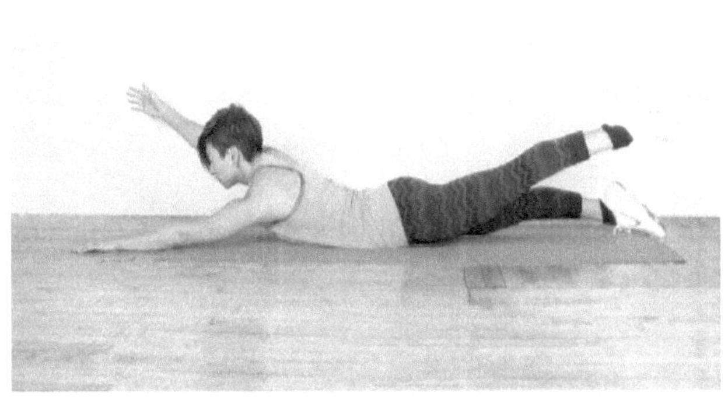

a. Lie facedown stretching your arms out and ensuring your palms face each other.
b. Lift one arm from the floor, keep it straight; also, your head and torso should equally be kept still.
c. Hold the position for a while and then bring your arm lower.
d. Repeat same on the other arm
e. You can also attempt lifting the leg opposite then raised arm a few inches away from the floor simultaneously.

26. Handstand push-up

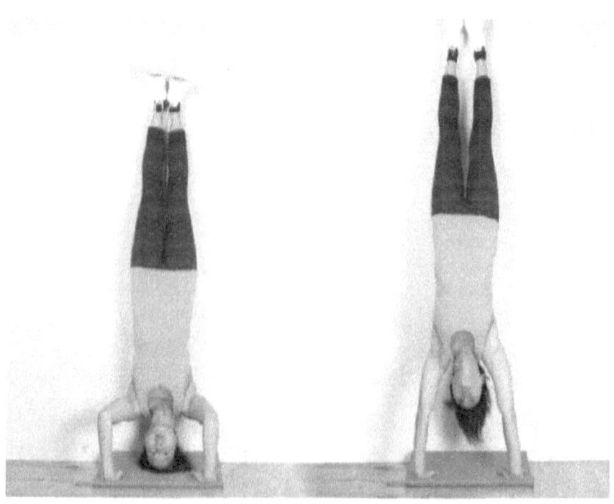

a. The headstand push is advisable for professional only.

b. First, get a mat and get into a handstand position done against the wall.

c. Now bend/move your elbows slightly to 90° angle,

d. Down do an upside-down push-up reverting your head to the floor and resting your legs against the wall.

27. Judo push-up:

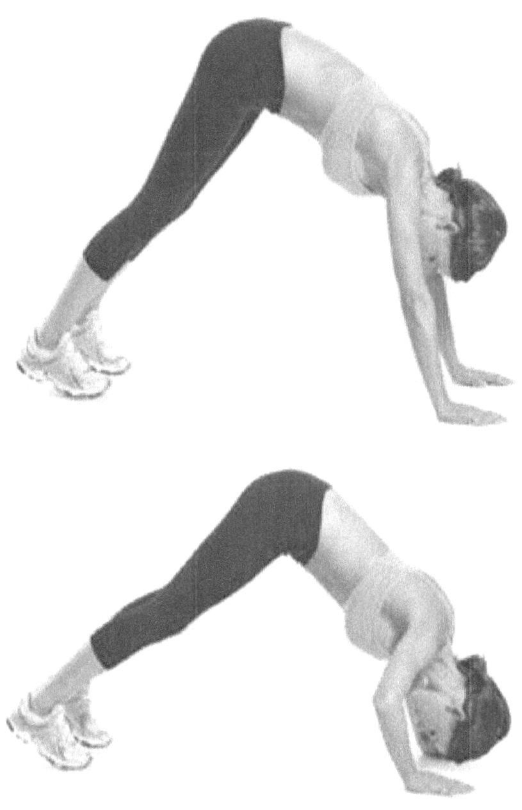

a. While in a push-up position, lift your hips and then lower font of your body using your hands, continue till your chin is close to the floor.
b. Lift your head and shoulders while lowering your hips and keeping your knees away from the floor.
c. Complete the move by returning your hip to being raised, and then repeat for 30-60 sec.

28. Superman

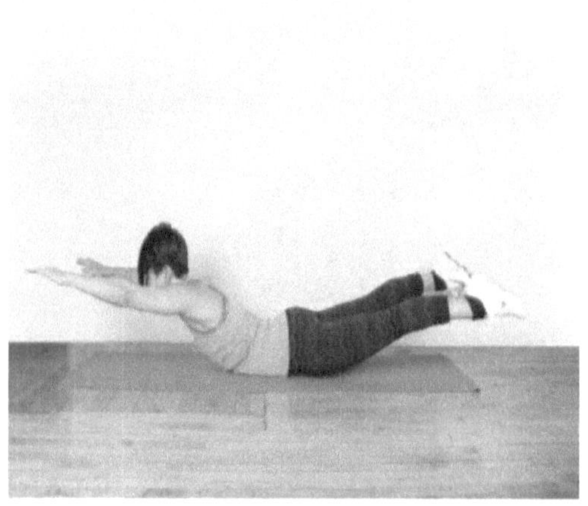

a. Lie face down, extending your arms and legs forward.

b. Keep your torso still while raising your arms and legs at the same time, to form a small back curve.

29. Standard push-up

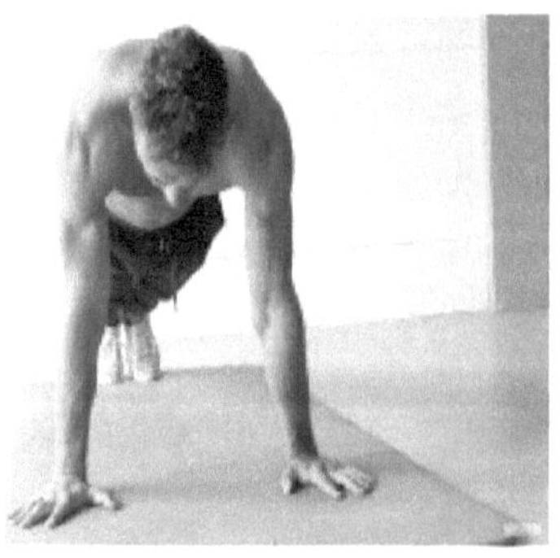

a. Lie flat on the floor; place your hands shoulder-width away from each other.

b. Ensure your feet are spaced at a hip distance while at the same time, tightening your core.

c. Slightly bend your elbows until your chest touches the floor
and immediately push back up.

d. Throughout the work-out, ensure your elbow is kept close to
your body.

30. Plyometric Push-up:

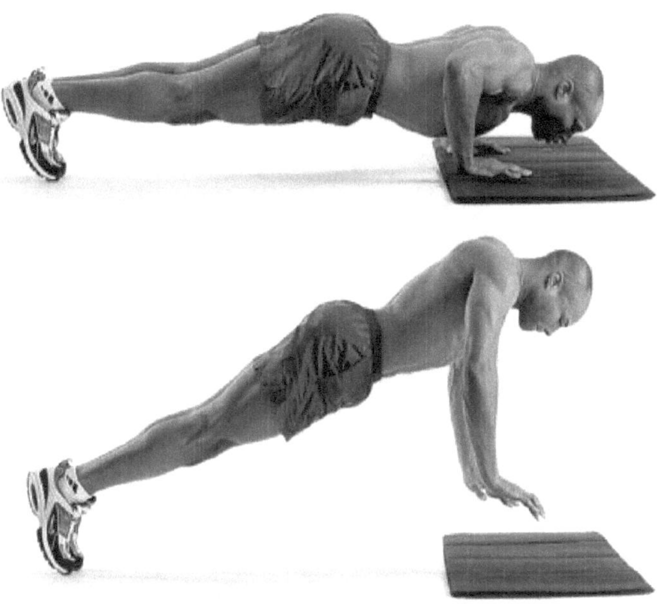

a. Do this on a mat, starting with a push-up.

b. Take a jump by pushing up hard, such that your hands

leave the floor and your hand in the air for about 5

secs or more.

c. Land back on the mat with your hands and repeat the

motion.

31. Donkey kick

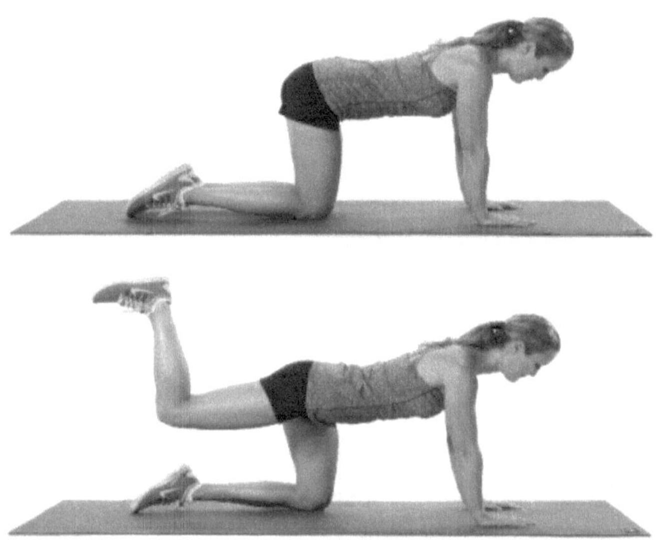

a. Begin in a push up position holding your legs
together.

b. Tighten your core kicking your legs into the air and
bending your knees and also moving your feet back.

c. Ensure you land gently when you're returning to your
starting position.

32. Rotational push-up

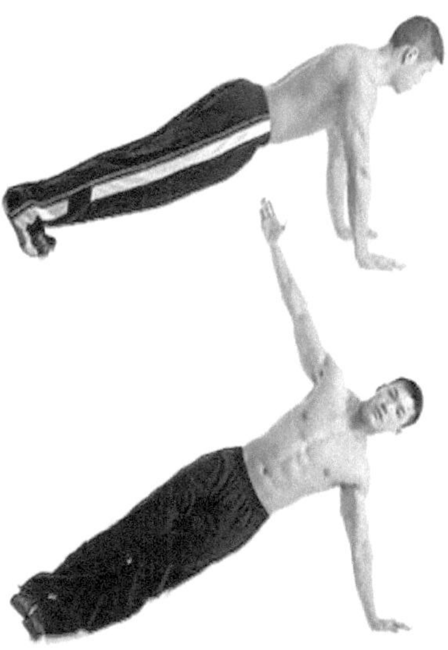

a. Start with a push up position, and then rotate your body towards the right.

b. Move your hand over your head to form a T shape using your arms and torso.

c. Return to your starting position, repeat the pushup and rotate body to the left.

33. Reverse fly

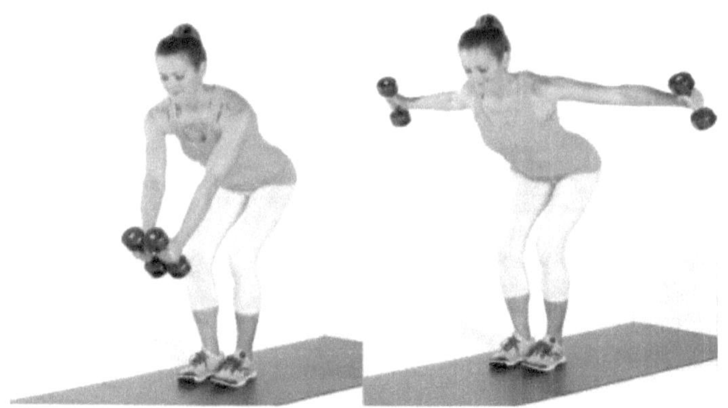

a. Begin by standing straight, placing one foot in front of the other and then bend front knee slightly.

b. Face both palms together and engage your abs

c. From your waist region slightly bend forward extending your arms out to the sides and then squeeze your shoulder blades

Chapter 11

Calisthenics exercise for shoulder and arms

34. Boxer

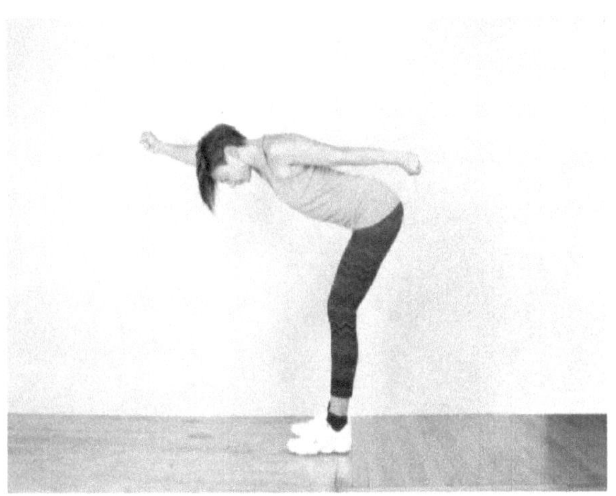

a. Begin by taking a standing position with your knee bent and your feet apart by hip-width.

b. Now continually bend forward until your upper body (torso) is nearly parallel in position to the floor.

c. Tuck elbows in, while extending one of your arms forward and extending the other one backwards.

d. After a while, swap the arms.

35. Diamond push-up

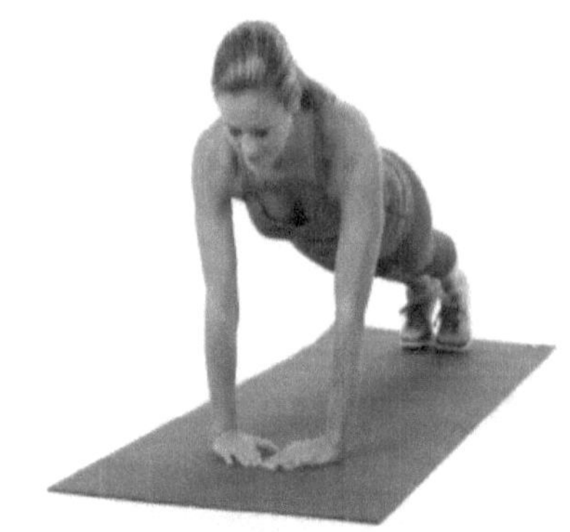

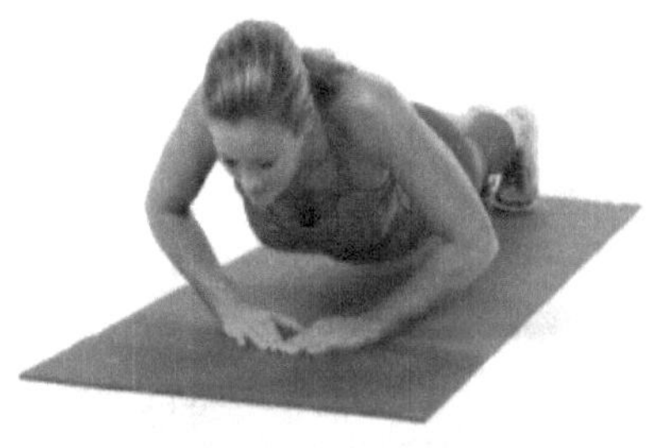

a. Begin with a standard push up position

b. Place your hands such that it forms a diamond shape (touch
    your thumbs and your index finger together to form the
    shape) and then continue your push-ups.

36. Arm circling

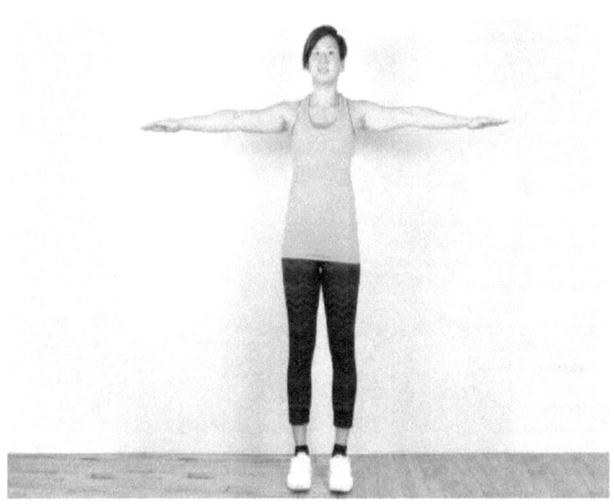

a. Taking a standing position with your arms stretched out at both sides, perpendicular to the upper body,

b. Make clockwise circles slowly, doing 1 foot in diameter for about 20-30 secs.

c. Reverse your motion and go anticlockwise.

37. Triceps dip

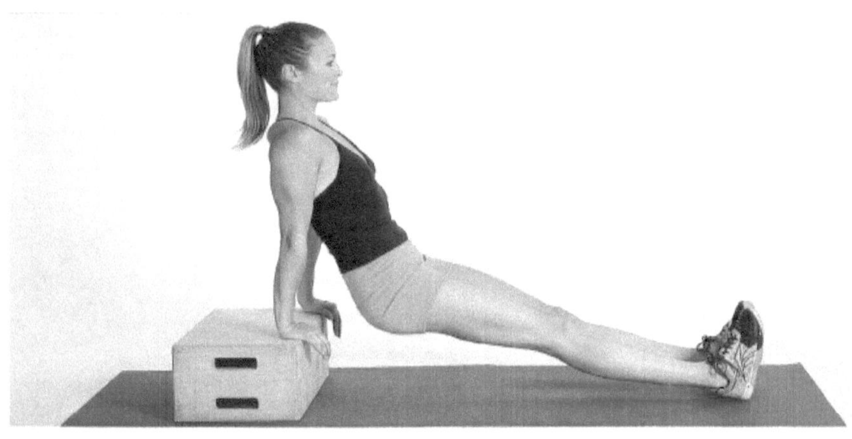

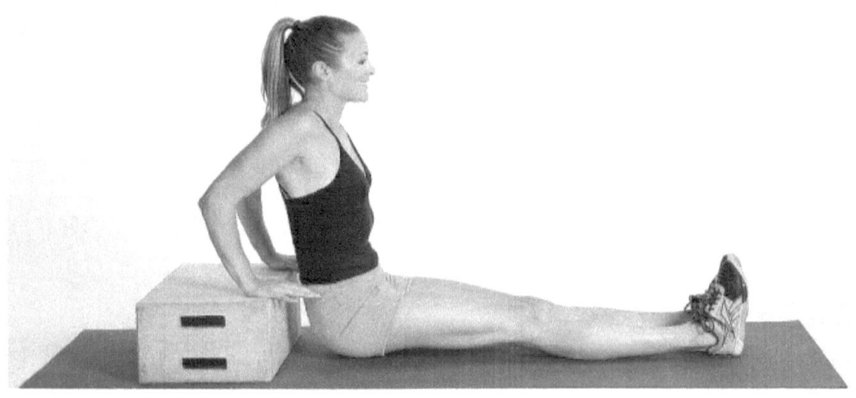

a. Sit on the ground or a mat, close to a bench, and ensure your knees are bent slightly.

b. Now grab the edge of the bench (elevated surface) and straighten your arms.

c. Bend your hands by angle 90° and straighten your arms again, while pushing your heels into the floor.

d. You can also try lifting your left leg while reaching your right arm to grab the bench.

Chapter 12

Calisthenics exercise for core strengthening

38. Bicycle

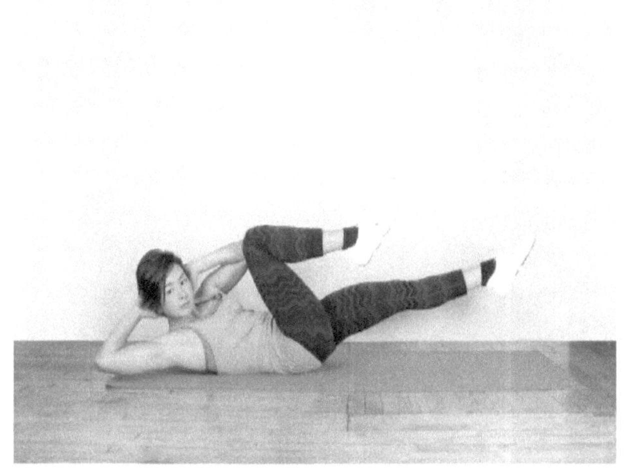

a. Lie flat on a mat face up, bending your knees and placing your hands behind your head.

b. Now bring the bent knee in towards your chest.

c. Move your right elbow towards your left knee and at the same time strengthen your right leg.

d. Now continue as though pedaling a bicycle; alternating your legs and hands.

39. Sprinter sit-up

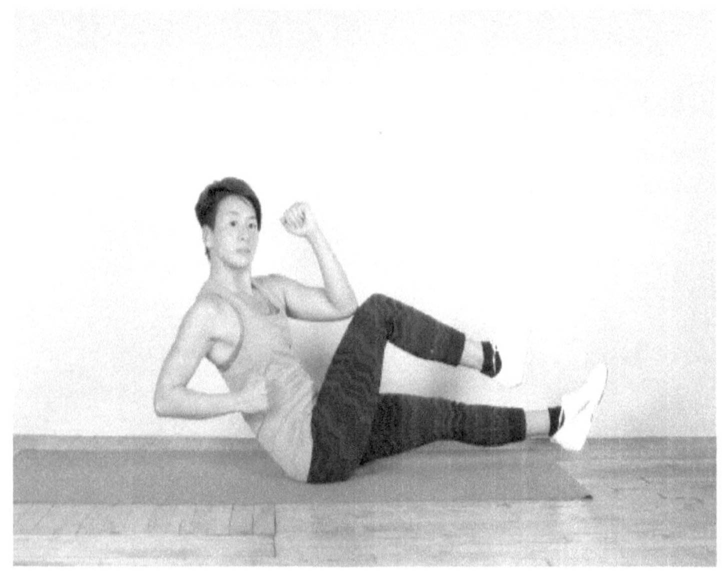

a. Lie flat with your face up, strengthen your legs.

b. Place arms by the sides and elbows bent by 90°.

c. Sit up as you bring your right elbow down towards your left knee.

d. Now return to your starting position and repeat the process alternating your elbows and knees.

40. Shoulder bridge

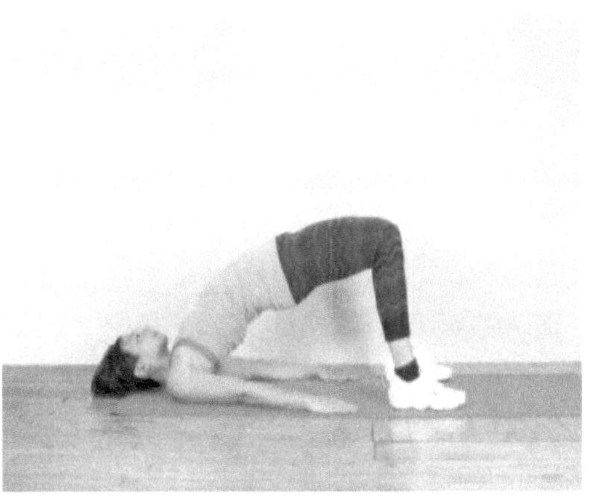

a. Lie flat with face-up, bending your knees and keeping your feet apart by your hip-width.

b. Place your arms sideways and slowly lift your spine as well as your hips. Leave your head, feet, shoulders and arms on the floor.

c. Now, slowly lift one leg while increasing the pressure on your core.

d. Bring your leg down slowly and lift it again, do as many reps as you can, before lowering your spine to the floor again.

41. Hollow Body Hold:

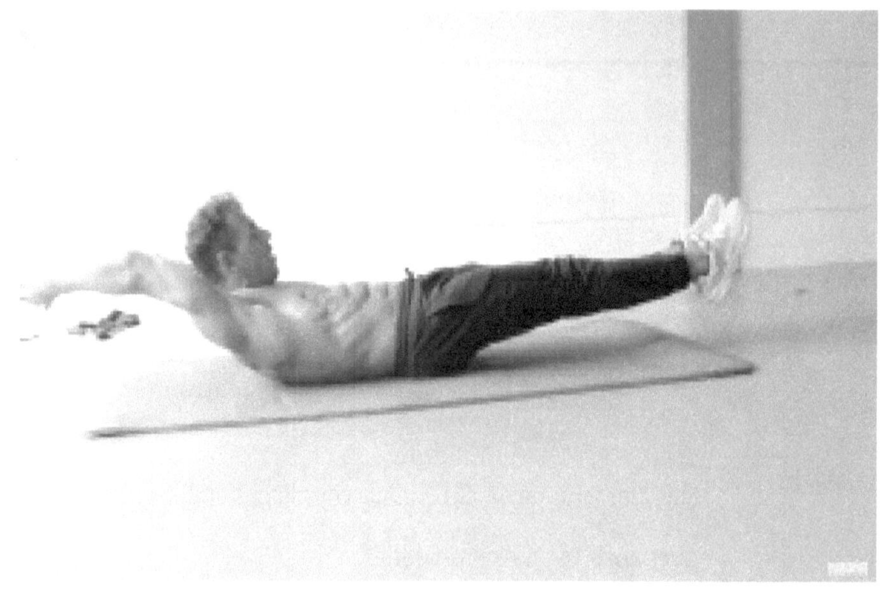

a. Lie flat on the floor face up.
b. Now lift your legs and scapula in the air at the same time,
c. Hold that position for about 30 secs or as long as you can

42. Flutter kick

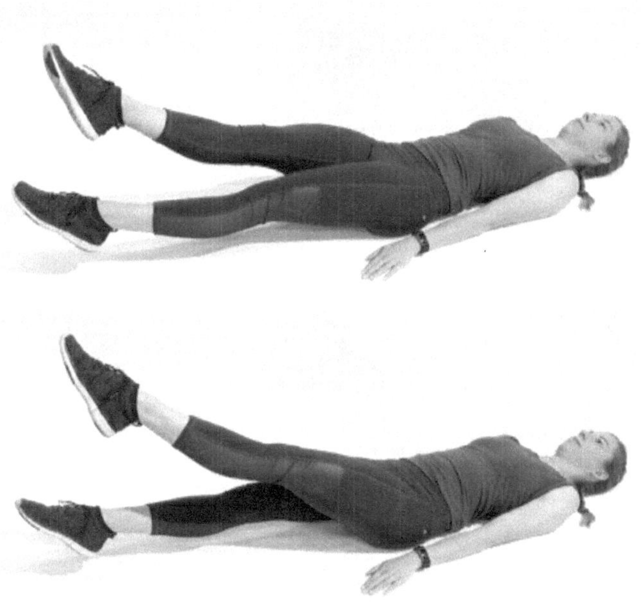

a. Lie flat with face-up, arms positioned at your sides and your palms facing down.
b. Extend your legs and lift heels about 5 inches up off the floor.
c. Now begin kicking your legs up and down while you also keep your core actively engaged.
d. Continue for about a minute.

43. CRUNCH:

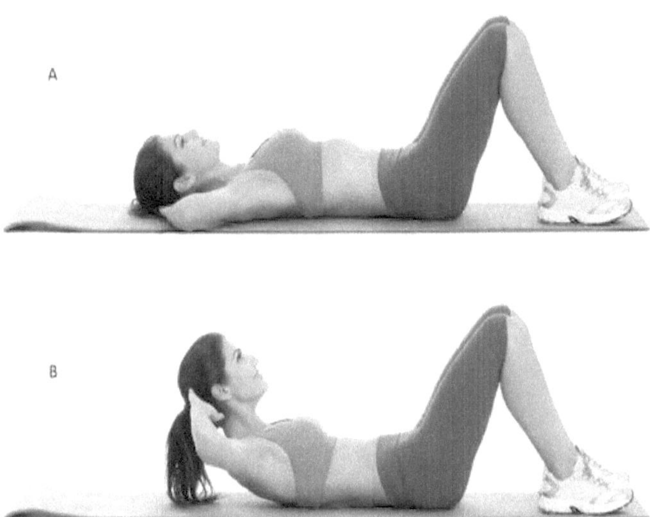

a. Lie facing up, bending your knees and keeping your feet flat against the floor.
b. Place your hands behind your head and then slightly lower your chin.
c. Lift your head and shoulder off the floor in other to engage your core,
d. Continue lifting it up until your torso is off the ground and then lower it back again and repeat the motion.

44. Dynamic prone plank

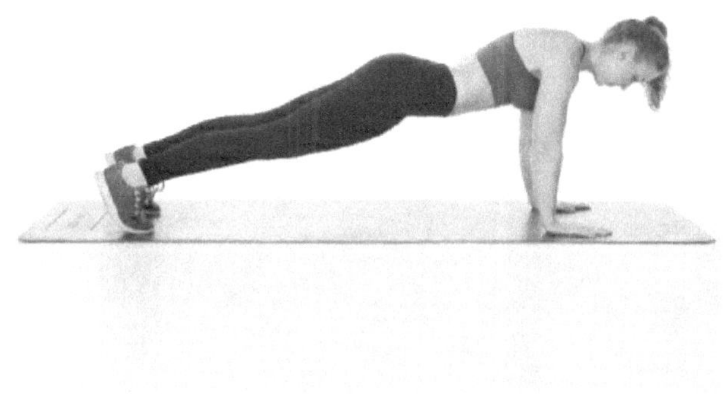

a. Start by taking a plank position,

b. Raise hips as high as possible and lower them back

immediately.

c. Continue the motions ensuring your back remains

straight.

45. Side plank

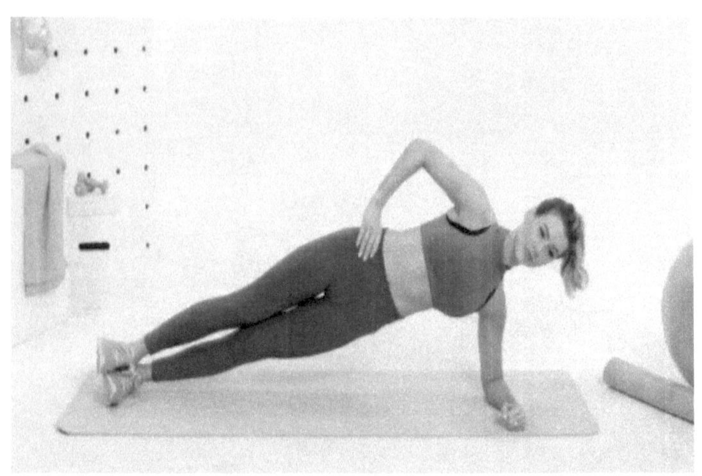

a. Lie flat face up and then roll to either side of your body,

b. Lift your body weight onto one foot and elbow

c. Ensure your hips are also lifted, and your core is actively engaged.

d. Maintain that position for 30-60 secs or as long as you can.

46. Segmental rotation

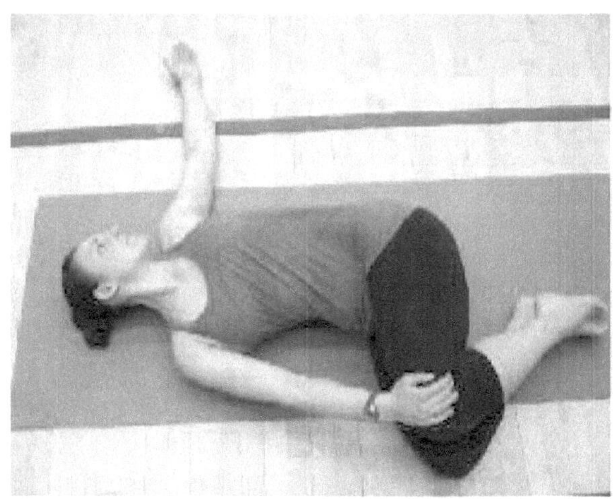

a. Lie flat face up, bending your knees and tightening your core.

b. Gradually let your knees fall gently to the left, giving you a good stretch.

c. Sustain the position for a while.

d. Return your legs to the centre and then repeat the action on the right side of your body, continue alternating between the sides.

47. L seat

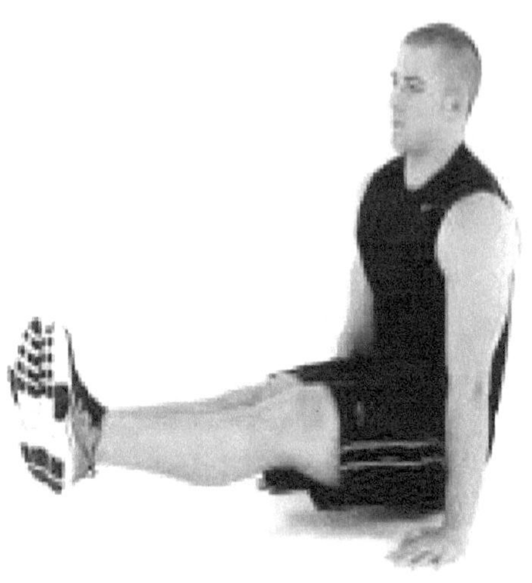

a. Begin by sitting with your legs extended out and flex your
    feet also.

b. Keep your hands on the floor and round your torso slightly.

c. Next, raise up your hips from the floor and hold it that way
    for about 5 seconds and then relax the hip.

d. Repeat the motion for a while.

48. Russian twist.

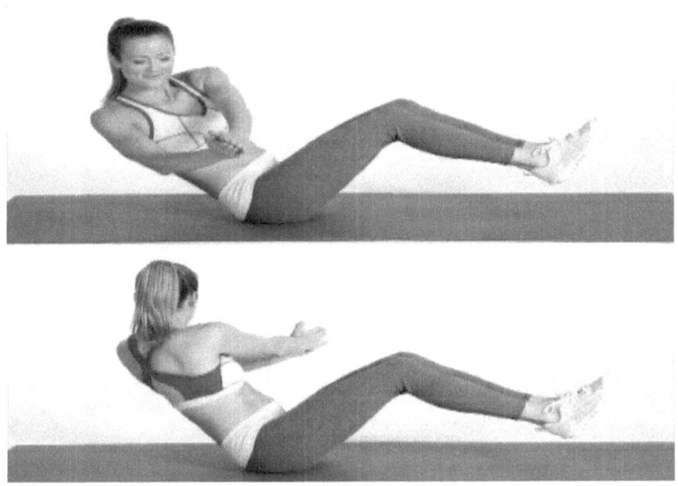

a. Start by sitting on the floor bending your knees and feet together while you lift it a few inches away from the floor.

b. Hold your back at angle 45° to the floor moving your arms from side to side while twisting it.

c. Continue the twisting motion slowly.

49. Single-leg abdominal press

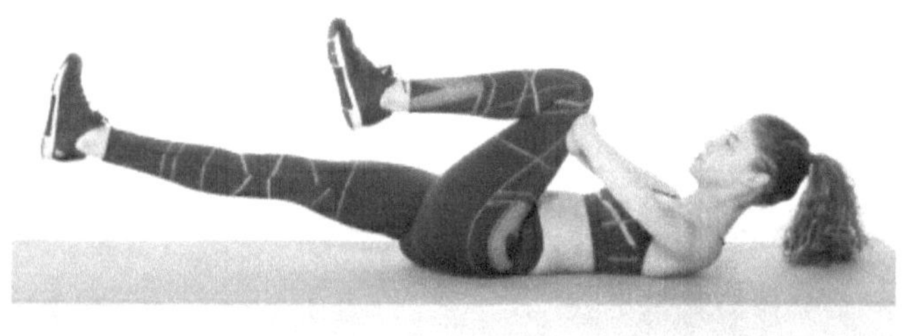

a. Lie with face up, bending your knees and keeping your feet flat on the floor.

b. Tighten your core and lift your right leg up while bending your knee to at 90° angle.

c. Push your right hand forward and place it on your lifted knee, tightening your core in order to create pressure between your knee and hand.

d. Hold that position for 5 secs and bring your back lower.

e. Alternate to left hand and knee.

50. Double-leg abdominal press

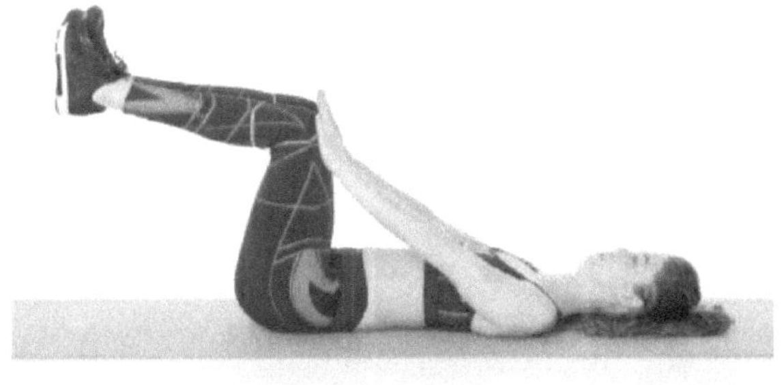

a. Follow the same process above, but instead use your two legs.

b. Put both legs up together and push your hands against your knees.

Chapter 13

How get rid of body fat

Ok, so you want to get rid of body fats and cruise that muscled body with magnificent packs on display, then you should read on. In this chapter, we'll look at some things you could do to burn off the fat.

What is Shredding?

This refers to the process of losing belly fat, burning off any excess that does not suit you and develop your body to the physique that you want or desire.

Some persons begin by dieting without building up the muscles underneath their flesh, and hence they turn out looking all small. You must first realize that weight loss is a gradual process and does not happen overnight; you must learn to be consistent and follow through with whatever path you choose in taking down the belly fats.

For a lot of persons, shredding entails building muscle mass first before they focus on losing fat. That being said, focusing on one alone would not help in any way, this could take months or even years, but with consistency, you'll be able to track the difference. So we'll be looking at how you can achieve both.

1. Build Muscle:

    Yes, you must burn fat, but then it is equally important you build the muscle underneath. It should be noted that more muscle mass translates to higher calorie needs, and hence you weigh more, although you look lean because muscles take up less space than fat; this is known as lean body mass.

    Don't forget that abs is muscles and increasing and strengthening the abs size can help give the required definition to your stomach. So you should be involved in core exercises majorly, but mixing with another form of exercises. Core exercises include;

    a. Planks
    b. Sit-ups

c. Oblique twists
d. Leg lifts
e. Flutter kicks

2. Cut down Calories consumption:

Alongside exercising, it is equally vital you control your intake
of calories. But do not cut it too low.
Calories work in such a way that they provide 100% of needed
body energy daily, and so when you take in more than you need
per day, they are stored as an energy reserve in the form of fats.
And then if you eat less, you're your body taps into this reserve
and burn the fat off. Hence this is the most effective method to
control calories.

3. Consume enough protein:

Increasing your protein intake, as it would help supply the
nutrients to build, repair and also maintain your lean tissue. It
equally helps to protect your lean muscle in case of a calorie
deficit; hence you lose more body fat and not lean muscle.

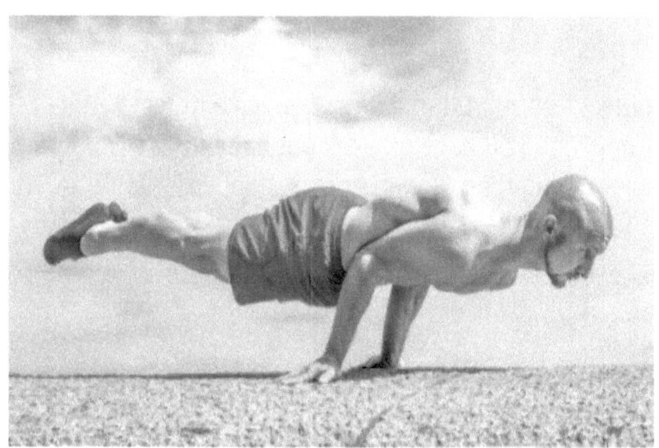

Chapter 14

How to move from beginners to intermediate and then expert in calisthenics

Often time this is a question you find beginners asking, either at the beginning of their calisthenics work out or some weeks into it. Everyone wants to be doing the big stuff and develop a killer body, but then we must remember that Rome was not built in a day.

However, if moving to intermediate level quickly is your goal right now, then I'm sure you'd find this helpful as I'll be looking at some hacks that could help answer your question.

Determine the reason you started calisthenics:

This is very important as the reason would sustain you through the days. So if your reason is to feel more energetic, flexible and more in tune with your mind and body, then you're obviously on the right track. It's also easier to continue in the practice if you develop a love for it, as this would spur you to try out new things that would help you reach your goal.

Start by taking baby steps:

Yes, as I said before, Rome was not built in a day. You have to realize that calisthenics is like a journey, one you have to work out patiently. Ensure you warm up, and also you cool down, these are all crucial steps that would teach you discipline as you go further.

Set goals:

This is equally important before you start calisthenics, you have to make certain your goals, and note them down. This would spur you to do better so you can meet your deadlines.

Keep track of your progress:

Doing this would be easy if you have goals set already. Have a book/journal, where you record your achievements daily or weekly. This way, you know how far you've gone in actualizing your goals.

Consistency:

It's not enough to start and continue on the days you feel like, no, to achieve your goals, you have to be consistent. Ensure you give your body a good challenge, keep increasing your reps and sets as you continue.

Rest when needed:

As much as it's good to keep pushing yourself, it's also advisable you rest as much as possible. When you feel aches and pain that's a sign that you should take a well-deserved rest.

Learn from others:

As a beginner, there's so much you don't know. But all these you could learn from others by asking questions. Never be too proud to solicit for help when you need, this way you grow fast.

You could follow a beginner's routine timetable and then move to intermediate on the completion of the beginners' duration. But then, without the points mentioned above, it would all be a waste. But if you can combine that alongside a manual, then you're steps away from getting your muscles and packs.

www.ingramcontent.com/pod-product-compliance
Lightning Source LLC
Chambersburg PA
CBHW020133180726
47992CB00022B/2927